Keto Bread

The Easy to Follow Ketogenic Cookbook for Your Low-Carb Diet with 40 Wheat and Gluten-Free Recipes. Enjoy Delicious Muffins, Cookies, Buns, Bagels, Bread Loaves, Pizza Crusts, & Breadsticks

Amanda Jason

© Copyright 2019 by Amanda Jason —All rights reserved.

This eBook is provided with the sole purpose of providing relevant information on a specific topic for which every reasonable effort has been made to ensure that it is both accurate and reasonable. Nevertheless, by purchasing this eBook you consent to the fact that the author, as well as the publisher, are in no way experts on the topics contained herein, regardless of any claims as such that may be made within. As such, any suggestions or recommendations that are made within are done so purely for entertainment value. It is recommended that you always consult a professional prior to undertaking any of the advice or techniques discussed within.

This is a legally binding declaration that is considered both valid and fair by both the Committee of Publishers Association and the American Bar Association and should be considered as legally binding within the United States.

The reproduction, transmission, and duplication of any of the content found herein, including any specific or extended information will be done as an illegal act regardless of the end form the information ultimately takes. This includes copied versions of the work both physical, digital and audio unless express consent of the Publisher is provided beforehand. Any additional rights reserved.

Furthermore, the information that can be found within the pages described forthwith shall be considered both accurate and truthful when it comes to the recounting of facts. As such, any use, correct or incorrect, of the provided information will render the Publisher free of responsibility as to the actions taken outside of their direct purview. Regardless, there are zero scenarios where the original author or the Publisher can be deemed liable in any fashion for any damages or hardships that may result from any of the information discussed herein.

Additionally, the information in the following pages is intended only for informational purposes and should thus be thought of as universal. As befitting its nature, it is presented without assurance regarding its prolonged validity or interim quality. Trademarks that are mentioned are done without written consent and can in no way be considered an endorsement from the trademark holder.

Table of Contents

Introduction 1

Chapter 1: Ingredients, Keto Bread Essentials, and Tools You Need for Your Keto Breads 3

   Ingredients 3

      Butters 3

      Flours 4

      Sweeteners 6

      Other Essentials 7

   Keto Bread Essentials 8

      Cookies 8

      Bagels 9

      Bread Loaves 9

   Tools You Need 10

Chapter 2: Methods to Follow the Keto Diet and Keep Low Amount of Carbs 13

   Methods to Follow the Keto Diet 13

   Keep Low Amount of Carbs 14

   Nutritional Information Note for This Cookbook 17

Chapter 3: Time and Money Saving Tips 18

   Time-Saving Tips 18

   Money Saving Tips: 20

Chapter 4: Muffin Recipes 23

   Blueberry Muffins 23

   Chocolate Chip Muffins 25

   Cinnamon Sugar Muffins 27

   Double Chocolate Muffins 29

   Egg Muffins 31

French Toast Muffins 32

Pumpkin Cream Cheese Muffins 33

Raspberry Lemonade Muffins 35

Chapter 5: Cookie Recipes 36

Chocolate Sea Salt Cookies 36

Coconut Cookies 38

Florentine Cookies 40

Nutty Cookies 42

Nutty Chocolate Chip Cookies 43

Oatmeal Cookies 45

Oreo Cookies 47

Vanilla Crescent Cookies 49

Chapter 6: Bun and Bagel Recipes 51

Bun Recipes 51

    Dinner Rolls 51

    Hawaiian Sweet Rolls 53

    Mini Buns 55

    Sesame Buns 56

Bagel Recipes 58

    Blueberry Cheesecake Bagels 58

    Cheese Bagels 60

    Jalapeno Bagels 62

    Pizza Bagel Bites 64

Chapter 7: Bread Loaf Recipes 66

Blueberry Bread Loaf 66

Cauliflower Bread Loaf 68

Cheese and Bacon Bread Loaf 70

Hearty Seeded Bread Loaf 72

Pumpkin Bread Loaf 74

Quick Low-Carb Bread Loaf 77

Savory Bread Loaf 79

Chapter 8: Pizza Crust and Breadstick Recipes 81

Pizza Crust Recipes 81

Coconut Flour Pizza Crust 81

Fathead Pizza Crust 83

Zero Carb Pizza Crust 84

Breadstick Recipes 86

Cauliflower Breadsticks.. 86

Cheese Breadsticks 88

Garlic Breadsticks 90

Italian Breadsticks 92

Rosemary Sea Salt Breadsticks... 94

Zucchini Breadsticks 96

Index for the Recipes 98

Chapter 4: Muffin Recipes 98

Chapter 5: Cookie Recipes 98

Chapter 6: Bun and Bagel Recipes 98

Chapter 7: Bread Loaf Recipes 99

Chapter 8: Pizza Crust and Breadstick Recipes 99

Introduction

Congratulations on downloading your copy of the *Keto Bread: The Easy to Follow Ketogenic Cookbook for Your Low-Carb Diet with 40 Wheat and Gluten-Free Recipes. Enjoy Delicious Muffins, Cookies, Buns, Bagels, Bread Loaves, Pizza Crusts, & Breadsticks.* I'm delighted that you have chosen to take this avenue to incorporate the Keto diet plan in your life.

Whether you are new to the Keto diet or have been testing out the dishes for years, the recipes, tricks, and tips you'll find here will help you prepare a healthy variety of bread that will make your mouth water. The plan goes by many different names such as the low-carb diet, the Keto diet, and the low-carbohydrate diet & high-fat (LCHF) diet plan. But we will keep it simple and call it the Keto diet in this cookbook.

The recipes in this book are easy to make and do not take that much time as we know that it is important to everybody. There are money and time-saving tips inside that will help you to integrate the Keto diet pretty easily into your life as you will be able to make most of these recipes ahead of time.

The recipes that you will find inside will not only satisfy your rumbling stomach but also make you feel good that you are taking this step towards a healthier life. We hope that this cookbook helps to show you the world of possibilities with the Keto diet.

Some of the recipe items may require a few more steps, but each recipe will provide you with an estimated preparation and cooking time, amount of servings, and a list of nutritional values including calories, net carbohydrates, protein, and fats. It is all laid out for you in a simple to follow list of instructions to get started on incorporating the Keto diet in your life today.

There are plenty of books on Keto diet in the market today and thanks again for choosing this one! Every effort was made to ensure that it is full of as much useful information as possible.

Chapter 1: Ingredients, Keto Bread Essentials, and Tools You Need for Your Keto Breads

Ingredients

There are some main ingredients that are necessary for the Keto diet to have the high-fat content that you need instead of the carbs. You will find that these ingredients will be the new staple in your pantry, and here you will find out why these substitutes for your normal diet will not leave you dissatisfied. In fact, your body will thank you.

Butters

Cashew butter is a substitute for traditional butter that gives your dishes a sweet flavor naturally. It also helps your sweet treats to have a more rich and creamy dough. You may choose between 100% cashew butter and some varieties which have sunflower oil included. Note that the butter with sunflower oil will add a more-oily consistency to your sweet recipes, and they will be denser.

Coconut oil can be used in substitute in these recipes instead of butter. This is a good choice for people who had a lactose intolerance or dairy allergy.

Grass-fed butter has been shown to have higher contents of nutrients such as linoleic acid (CLA) and loaded with beneficial fats and vitamins versus traditional butter which generally comes from GMO fed cows. Grass-fed butter also contains a dominant anti-inflammatory fat called butyric acid and anti-oxidants which aid in your overall health.

Flours

Almond flour is quite popular in the Keto diet as the main substitute for the traditional wheat flours. It has a much higher fat content than wheat flour which tends to burn recipes much quicker. You will find that many of the oven temperatures in these recipes are lower than the traditional recipes for that very reason.

Because almond flour is made just from almonds, you can make it right in your kitchen. All that you are going to need is a blender that is high-powered to pulverize the almond. The benefits of almond flour are that it is filled with heart-healthy fats and is naturally gluten-free, making it the number one choice in the Keto diet.

There are many other benefits to almond flour that will make you fall in love with it while you get acquainted with the Keto diet. It has been shown to manage healthy levels of blood sugar along with improving heart health. Improving energy levels and helping with weight loss, you cannot deny that almond flour is going to become your new pal in the kitchen.

As a rule of thumb, when you are converting old-fashioned recipes, you should use 50% more almond flour versus the amount of traditional wheat flour.

Coconut flour has extremely high levels of saturated fats (which are healthy for you!), and these fats actually aid in metabolism and assist in balancing out the blood sugar levels naturally. Coconut flour has many other benefits such as being high in fiber and low in carbs and sugar and is absolutely packed with vitamins and minerals.

Even though it is more expensive (See Chapter 3 for the money saving tips!), it does not take much of this flour to go a long way in these recipes. There are smaller amounts needed for the Keto diet recipes compared to almond flour as it is much more absorbent, and it fills you up more than traditional wheat flour. Because coconut flour is more absorbent, you will find that those recipes will require more butter and eggs. The taste of the coconut flour also compliments many fruity dishes as well.

The reason why everyone loves coconut flour is that it aids your body to maintain healthy blood sugar levels and keeps them more stable. And as we said, it makes you feel fuller, so you will not be wanting to grab unneeded snacks during the day. Although you still may want to after seeing the treats that we have in store for you!

Coconut flour actually improves digestive health as well, keeping everything working on a regular cycle. This is because it has five times more fiber as compared to the fiber levels in traditional wheat flour.

The metabolism benefits for coconut flour also offer quick energy as it contains medium-chain fatty acids (MCTs). These are healthy fats that help you to get up and going to keep burning off the fat.

And the benefits of coconut flour continue. It actually keeps you to stay healthier by protecting your body because of the antiviral and antibacterial properties it contains. And, if you have a nut allergy, coconut flour is your best friend as you can use it for all of your baking needs without the worry of an allergic reaction.

Two brands that are recommended are the Nutiva and Coconut Secret brands flour. That is if you do not decide to make it in your kitchen yourself.

Sweeteners

There is a wide variety of sweeteners available for Keto diet followers. We use Swerve throughout the book for most of the recipes because it is one of the top approved brands of sweetener for the Keto diet. It is also sugar-free! However, it is up to personal preference which sweetener you use.

Monk fruit sweetener is also a popular choice. You must know that this sweetener will make your dishes sweeter versus the other choices of sweeteners. However, the people who do prefer monk fruit sweetener find that other sweeteners have a cooling effect and bad aftertaste. If you find this to be true, this will be the choice in sweeteners for you.

Swerve has the same amount of sweetness compared to traditional white sugars found in recipes. It measures out to be the same if converting recipes after you get deeper into the world of keto, as you will find yourself going through your grandmother's recipes to convert them. There are also no calories in this sweetener, so it will help you to not feel guilty when you are eating those keto cookies.

Truvia is the brand name for the natural sweetener of the stevia plant. Most people who are into eating healthy have heard of stevia, or the common name is erythritol. This is a sugar alcohol that is found in melons and grapes and also has no calories. Many people say that there is a metallic taste to stevia, but others compare it to the same taste as traditional sugar. Again, experiment with the sweeteners to find what suits your palate.

As a note, if you have been diagnosed with autoimmune disorders or a leaky gut, it may actually have ill effects for your digestive system. If you suffer from these disorders or are allergic to corn, consult your doctor about which sweetener is best for your personal diet.

You can use granulated sweeteners in place of confectioner sweeteners. If you do substitute the granulated sweeteners, you will find that you will be able to feel the texture of the granules in your sweet treats. The confectioner sweeteners do work best in the sweet recipes, but it is up to your personal preference.

Other Essentials

Fresh organic eggs are recommended versus the eggs you buy in the carton from your grocery store. This is due to them usually containing MSG, and the packaging companies are not required to label this on the packaging. If you want to stay true to the keto lifestyle, switch to the fresh organic egg option.

Organic eggs are high in phosphatidylcholine which keeps the nervous system in the brain functioning at optimal levels. They are also high in protein, anti-oxidants, and vitamin E, so you really cannot go wrong when you make the switch.

Mozzarella cheese is a key ingredient in many of the keto recipes, especially the Fathead Bread. There are loads of nutrients in mozzarella cheese including riboflavin, protein, phosphorus, and biotin.

Xanthan gum is used in particular with the cookie recipes to keep the cookies from crumbling, and it actually makes the cookies softer and tastier. It is usually an optional ingredient, but experiment with this ingredient, and you may find that you cannot live without it.

Keto Bread Essentials

There are many tips in helping you with these recipes and others that you find along your journey into the Keto diet. Here are some basic cooking tips for this cookbook that you will find helpful for the different types of recipes.

Cookies

If you prefer to have crispy cookies while you try out these Keto diet delights, be sure to make sure to **let the cookies cool completely**, even if this means overnight. They will be less crumbly, and you will not regret every crunch in your mouth.

If you prefer sweeter cookies, add 1/4 tsp **stevia glycerite** to any of the recipes to appease your sweet tooth.

If you find that you are not getting the fluffiness that you desire in your cookies, add half a TSP of **apple cider vinegar** into the ingredients. It will alter the cookie texture, but it will give the cookies more rise.

Bagels

Nut flours make a denser bagel and as such, you may want to substitute your own homemade or store-bought nut flours. On the other hand, almond flour creates a fluffier and light bagel, so use the ingredient that will give you the bagel that you most prefer.

Bread Loaves

When you whip the **egg whites** in any bread loaf recipe, it will help the bread to rise and results in a more light and airy loaf of bread versus mixing the entire egg at once which creates a denser loaf of bread.

If you decide to go with the lighter bread loaf version, you need to use a food processor to whip the eggs until they are fluffy and light. Then add to the dough in small amounts until incorporated. If you overmix the egg whites into the dough, it will be the same result as if you mixed the entire egg at once.

Because of the substitution of gluten-free flours from old-fashioned recipes, you may find that the **bread loaves do not tend to rise** as much. One way to remedy this is to use a smaller pan to force the bread loaf to be taller. The downside to this is you will have a marginally higher carb count per serving and get fewer slices out of the bread.

Alternatively, you can use a combination of vinegar and baking soda which will cause a chemical reaction, producing carbon dioxide, which will naturally increase the volume of the batter. This will also get the desired effect of the bread loaf rising higher.

When baking your bread loaves, it is best to have all ingredients **non-refrigerated** before beginning. A tip to bring eggs to the correct temperature is to put them into a bowl of warm water for 3-4 minutes.

Put a portion of an aluminum foil on the pan's top during the last 15 mins. of baking if you find that the bread loaf is starting to **burn**.

Using fresh and new **baking powder** is essential in making sure you have the bread loaf that you are craving. You can test the freshness of the baking powder in your pantry by pouring 4 tablespoons of boiling water over 1/2 TSP of the baking powder. It is still good to use in your baking if it foams up immediately.

When you let the bread loaf cool in the pan, it will ensure it will not crumble to pieces when you cut the loaf into slices. This is especially true for the quick timed recipes.

Tools You Need

You will have many of these cooking utensils in your kitchen already, but if you collect these tools ahead of time, it will save you time, and you will have what you need to make the Keto diet a lifestyle change for you.

The items that you will need that you probably already own are the absolute basics for cooking and baking. These include basic **mixing bowls, electric mixer, stirring spoons, rolling pin**, and a **whisk**.

You will find that the **food processor** is a must-have in your kitchen, as it will help you to be able to bake these recipes much more quickly compared to mixing ingredients by hand.

When you are baking bread and sweets in the Keto diet, it is best to use **parchment paper** or **silicone-based pans and cooking trays** because they tend to stick to the pan more so than traditional recipes. The silicone products are brilliant when it comes to baking and especially with the Keto diet as nothing will be stuck to the silicone. When you decide to try the parchment paper liners, they also have the benefit of sweeties not getting too wet on the bottom.

The **Silpat** will make your life so much grander when it comes to rolling out the dough for the bread loaves and breadsticks. It is easy to wash, and nothing sticks to it. It is a good substitute for parchment paper, and it is reusable. The only downside is you cannot use sharp objects on the Silpat as it will cause it damage.

Cookie scoopers are a nice addition to the collection, as I can guarantee you will be using this tool a lot after tasting these recipes. It will help to keep your cookies in a uniform shape and makes baking much easier than scraping the dough off a spoon.

If you love the taste of brick oven pizzas, you can get this same effect with getting a **stone pizza pan** to cook the pizza crusts. This will make them extra crispy, and it is ideal if you enjoy super thin crust pizza. Using a stone pizza pan also allows for the pizza crust to cool even more quickly, so you can get to eat your healthy meal even faster.

All **ovens** heat differently depending on if they are along an outside wall of your home. Keep this in mind as you may need to raise or lower the oven temperature up or down by 25°F to get the desired time of baking.

Chapter 2: Methods to Follow the Keto Diet and Keep Low Amount of Carbs

Incorporating the recipes in this cookbook will certainly assist you in keeping in line with the guidelines of the Keto diet. The key to the Keto diet is to consume high fats and low carbs, but sometimes, this is tricky when you are just getting started. Here are some tips to assist you in making sure the transition into the lifestyle of Keto goes more smoothly for you.

Methods to Follow the Keto Diet

There is a lot of information out there as the Keto diet becomes more popular for weight loss, increasing your energy levels, improving overall mental clarity and moods, and even reversing Type 2 Diabetes.

The key information that is most important to remember on this diet is eliminating the foods you eat that are high in calories but less filling. These are the processed foods that most people in society eat because of time constraints or wanting some comfort food. Instead, focus on eating foods that are high in fiber and protein as they will be nutritious and more filling.

Because the Keto diet is a lifestyle change, you need to base your environment around you to support your new lifestyle choice. This means you will need to take a hard look at the food that you keep in your home.

When we feel we do not have any time or we are looking for creature comforts, usually we head to the kitchen. It would be best to do an inventory of what is in your pantry and get rid of anything that is not keto-friendly in your home. Believe me, once you bake the recipes we have for you, there will be no regrets about this decision.

You will find it will be a good change of habit to start planning your meals so that you can make sure that you have what you need when you are ready to bake. This also will be the case when you are traveling or working. Be sure to bring healthy snacks to eat in case you are not at home so that you will always be true to your new lifestyle.

You will also find the transition easier if you find other people who are doing just the same. There are groups that you can search online to hang out with people just like you. This will also be a good way to share ideas and build a support system to help you get over the hurdles of making any sort of lifestyle change will certainly bring.

Also keeping your eye on the final prize which it being healthier you will help you to achieve any of the health goals you are reaching for as it is a real possibility with the Keto diet. Whether it is needing to keep diabetes at bay, lowering inflammation, eliminating seizures, or you do not want unhealthy sugary processed foods to forever rule your life, all of these can be accomplished as long as you have the drive to do so.

Once you make the change, you will not look back.

Keep Low Amount of Carbs

As a general rule of thumb, you want to keep your total net carb count to 30 grams or less during the day, but you may find that you need to kick this up to 50 grams or even lower it to 20 grams depending on the activities you do during the day. This will kick your body into ketosis, making your body burn fat rather than carbs, which is what you want on the Keto diet. This same process occurs when you are fasting and actually aids in the glucose levels in the body to be naturally leveled-out.

The result of the Keto diet is weight loss due to the elimination of glucose from the body. When the body is turned into a fat burning machine, then this is when you will release the weight will start coming off. If you keep to the diets in the cookbook, then it will be an easy way to do just that.

The hardest challenge is keeping the count of your carbs low, but there are ways to accomplish this without causing too much stress.

The best way to keep a low amount of carbs during the Keto diet is to cut out all of the processed and sugary foods that you buy at the supermarket. This would also include sugary fruits such as bananas and oranges. Likewise, starchy foods high in carbs should be avoided. These are pasta, potatoes, rice, and bread.

On the other hand, when you add in vegetables such as cauliflower and broccoli, nuts, berries, and high-fat cheeses, you will find it easy to stay away from the carbs and still find success in the Keto diet.

Using the alternative ingredients in these recipes will actually make sure that you do not have to go without the foods you love and still live a healthy life.

Food tips to help with low carbs:

Even the pizzas in these recipes can pack in the carbs and calories. If you want to lower the amount you are taking, think about making mini pizzas instead of the full pizza crust. These are brilliant for snacks and can be frozen just the same and defrosted as a quick snack in less than 10 minutes.

Also, keep in mind that most of the carbs from pizza dishes come from the pizza dough itself. A way to remedy this is to pack more healthy vegetables and meats on the top to help keep you fuller for longer and you will not have the hit to your carb count for the day.

Flax Meal is a good alternative because it contains less net carbs and calories per serving. For example, if you were making the sesame bun recipe, it would be about 120 calories less per serving and have 3 less net carbs. If you are finding that you are not able to keep your carb intake at the recommended 30 grams or less a day, this is an option to consider.

Raw nuts are your best friend on the Keto diet as they are rich in fiber, anti-oxidants, vitamins, and healthy fats. They are a good on-the-go snack and have great benefits to your overall health. The following are the health benefits for adding raw nuts into your Keto diet.

- You lower your risk for diabetes
- Lowering your systolic blood pressure
- Stronger cardiovascular health
- Reduces your mortality risks
- Fewer risk factors for metabolic syndrome

As you can see, raw nuts are wonderful for people who are suffering from cardiovascular diseases, and many types of raw nuts will be able to help directly with those issues. This is because they contain an amino acid called L-arginine which helps with the overall health of the blood vessels and heart muscle.

Nutritional Information Note for This Cookbook

Nutritional information for the recipes provided is an approximate only. And substitutions that you use will alter the nutritional values and need to be personally researched to stay on track with the Keto diet. As such, we cannot guarantee the complete accuracy of the nutritional information given for any recipe in this cookbook. Erythritol carbs are not included in the net carb counts as it has been shown not to impact blood sugar. The method that net carbs are calculated is the total amount of carbs minus the fiber.

Chapter 3: Time and Money Saving Tips

In this day in age, we are always lacking in time and money. Well, the good news is you will not need to spend all day in the kitchen struggling to make a healthy meal for yourself and your family. In fact, this is probably going to change the more you get involved in the Keto diet lifestyle as you start seeing how your body looks healthier and you will feel it in your mind as well.

Time-Saving Tips

The biggest time-saving tip is you can double or even triple these recipes as they all keep for many days either on the counter or an even longer time in your freezer or refrigerator. It can't get easier than that!

If you are going to store your sweeties on the counter, keep them in an air-tight container as they will keep longer. As with the cookies, you can always keep them in the all familiar cookie jar as you know this always brings back wonderful memories of childhood. This method will also keep your sweet treats even softer.

Storing your keto sweets in the freezer or the refrigerator is just as easy. Simply wrap each pastry securely in plastic wrap, put them in a sealed container (only if putting into the refrigerator), or throw them into a zipping plastic bag. Whenever you need to eat them, you can put them inside the oven again to heat them up, throw them into the microwave, or even eat them straight out of the bag. This will make the cookies especially crispier, as you have already learned.

The method is quite similar for the bread loaves. Again, make sure they are completely cooled so you can slice them before you store them, or you can actually keep the bread loaves whole.

Whatever your preference is, know that the effect is the same as the sweeties. If you leave them out on the counter, the bread will stay softer and will keep for 2-3 days. If you put them in the freezer or refrigerator, they will become denser and will keep for up to one month. If you have stored the bread in the freezer, you can simply put it into the refrigerator a day before you want to serve.

The key before storing them away is to make sure that the sweets are completely cool beforehand. This will ensure that they will not end up crumbling to pieces and the excess moisture from the heat will not cause condensation on the packaging.

As for time-saving tips on the pizza crusts, a helpful tip when you are rolling out the dough is to use 2 pieces of parchment paper. One will go onto the counter, and the other will go on the top of the dough, creating a sandwich effect. This will ensure the rolling pin will not stick to the dough. This method is absolutely necessary for the fathead dough recipes as the dough has a sticky texture, but you can use it for any bread recipe that needs to be rolled and flattened.

You can even make pizza crusts in advance & place them into the fridge. Because they are so thin, you can pull them out an hour or two before you would like to have dinner. They will thaw nicely on the counter and then you just top with your favorite pizza ingredients and bake into the oven to heat the toppings. Now that is a quick dinner!

A time-saving tip for the cauliflower dishes which are found in the bread loaf and breadstick recipes is to prepare the cauliflower to be riced ahead of time. It will stay fresh in the refrigerator for 3 days before consuming and can be a great addition to any meal on its own.

The key is to make sure that as much moisture is removed as possible. If there is still juice present, it will make your bread loaf and breadsticks too soggy.

To do this, you will need an electric mixer to stir the cauliflower until it looks like crumbs. After this step is completed, you will then need to heat the cauliflower in a small cooking pot until tender. Then spoon the cauliflower in small amounts to a tea towel to squeeze and wring the water out. This step needs to be completed several times to make sure that all moisture content was removed.

Money Saving Tips:

You will find that the ingredients that are called for in the Keto diet recipes are going to be more expensive. Mentally, you will need to get past this fact because, again, you need to keep in mind why you have made the choice to begin this lifestyle change. Once you start seeing the benefits to your health, you will be hooked and try to find more ways to further your journey into this lifestyle change you have chosen.

Luckily, there are ways to ensure that you get the best bang for your buck when it comes to buying ingredients to stock your pantry. You will also find benefit in talking and researching on your own with what other people have found during their own personal journeys that it will help you on your own path.

One way to cut down costs is to make the almond and coconut flours in your own kitchen. As stated before, the almond flour can be made at home using a high-powered blender and buying almonds. This will also ensure the freshness of the final product, and you will feel even more empowered in your continued journey into the Keto diet.

If this seems overwhelming at first, then you can purchase these ingredients at local shops near you. Be sure to shop around for the best prices but know that the quality may vary. Read through the ingredients to make sure there are no other additives that are not specific to the keto diet and do not ever lose hope.

For instance, when you purchase the almond meal at the supermarket, it is going to be about $10 dollars for each pound. Do not fret! Many of these recipes call for smaller amounts compared to traditional recipes.

Alternatively, you can look on Amazon or other online shopping networks to have them delivered straight to your door without the hassle. Remember though to make sure the ingredients are in line with the Keto diet, and it will taste much healthier than the foods that you are accustomed to eating.

You can also look into other flour substitutes such as flax meal which has better benefits compared to almond flour. First off is the cost, as it will usually run you about $4 a pound compared to $10 a pound for the almond flour.

Costs for the coconut flour are considerably cheaper than almond flour, and you end up using less in the recipes. You can find several brands of coconut flour that will average about $5 per pound. Again, if you take advantage of the online shopping networks, you will have them delivered straight to you without the hassle of driving to several supermarkets to find the best price for your budget.

If you do not have a nut allergy, these would also be a good addition to your pantry and would substitute for the almond or coconut flours in the recipes. You will find that these nut flours will cost about $4 a pound as well.

Chapter 4: Muffin Recipes

Blueberry Muffins

Total Prep and Cooking Time: 30 minutes

Makes: 12 Muffins

Calories: 125, Protein: 6 g, Fat: 15 g, Net Carbs: 4 g

What you need:

½ cup of granulated sweetener Swerve

2 ½ cup of blanched almond flour

½ TSP of vanilla extract

¾ cup of blueberries

1 ½ TSP of baking powder—gluten-free

1/3 cup of almond milk, unsweetened

3 large eggs

¼ TSP of salt (optional)

1/3 cup of coconut oil—solid

Steps:

1. Make sure the stove to set to the temperature of 350°F. You need to line a standard cupcake pan with silicone muffin or baking paper liners.
2. Mix the baking powder, almond flour, salt, and sweetener in a big bowl used for mixing.
3. Use a smaller saucepan, on medium heat, heat the coconut oil then put it slowly to a mixture of flour when completely melted.

Then mix the eggs, unsweetened almond milk, & the extract of vanilla into the batter and combine completely.

4. When mixed thoroughly, carefully fold the blueberries into the mixture.

5. Distribute the batter to the muffin cups. Bake for a total of 20 mins. They will have a golden texture when completely baked.

Tricks and tips:

- Using frozen blueberries is acceptable for this recipe. A better recommendation is using fresh blueberries as the bread will be more uniform and less mushy.

- Separate the eggs for a lighter dough. See Chapter 3 under *Time-Saving Tips* for more details. When using this method, the blueberries need to be added last.

Chocolate Chip Muffins

Total Prep & Cooking Time: 30 minutes.
Makes: 12 Muffins
Calories: 88, Net Carbs: 2 g, Fats: 7 g, Protein: 2 g

What you need:

2 ounces of cream cheese
¼ cup of granulated Swerve sweetener
½ cup of coconut flour
1 tsp. of baking powder—gluten-free
4 T. of butter
¼ cup of sugar-free chocolate chips
3 large eggs
1/8 TSP of Xanthan gum
1 tsp. vanilla extract
¼ TSP of salt
1 cup of milk

Steps:

1. Set your stove to a temperature of 350°F. Line a small cupcake pan accompanied by silicone and baking paper muffin liners.
2. Mix the baking powder & coconut flour into the mixing bowl & swerve until combined.
3. Whip the butter, vanilla extract, and cream cheese until it becomes fluffy by using the stand mixer. Add one egg and mix. Repeat procedure until all eggs are mixed in thoroughly.

4. Combine the dry ingredients into the wet ingredient bowl slowly to make sure it is mixed well. Then in the bowl, pour off the milk and then mix it until incorporated fully. Fold the sugar free chocolate chips into the batter carefully.

5. Spoon or pour into the cupcake cups. Put it inside the oven for at least 18 to 20 mins. when the muffins' top turns brown.

Cinnamon Sugar Muffins

Total Prep & Cooking Time: 30 minutes.

Makes: 12 Muffins

Calories: 134, Net Carbs: 4 g, Fat: 26 g, Protein: 5 g

What you need:

For the muffin batter:

1 ½ cup almond flour—blanched

2 tsp. of baking powder—gluten-free

½ cup of confectioner Swerve sweetener

5 T. butter—softened

½ cup of heavy cream

1 TSP of vanilla

2 T. psyllium husk—pulverized

2 large eggs

1/2 TSP of ginger

1/2 TSP of allspice

1/2 TSP of nutmeg

For toppings:

1 TSP of cinnamon

2 T butter—melted

¼ cup Swerve sweetener—granulated

Steps:

1. Set the stove temperature to 350°F. Line a cupcake pan accompanied by silicone muffin baking paper cups.
2. Whip the confectioner sweetener, the butter, & the extract of vanilla in the medium-sized bowl approximately 5 mins. until it becomes a smooth consistency by the use of the electric mixer. Then beat the heavy cream and the eggs into the mixture.
3. In an additional medium mixing bowl, thoroughly whisk the remainder of the dry ingredients which include almond flour, psyllium husk powder, allspice, baking powder, ginger, and nutmeg, making sure the batter is smooth.
4. Then add the wet mixture slowly into the dry ingredient bowl while mixing continuously with the electric mixer to ensure it is combined.
5. Transfer the batter to the cups already prepared. Put the pan into the heated stove and bake it for 18 to 20 mins.
6. In the meantime, use a bowl and whisk together the granulated sweetener, cinnamon, and butter.
7. Use a spoon in dusting the muffins' topping while they are cooling so it melts into the muffins and serve them warm.

Double Chocolate Muffins

Total Prep & Cooking Time: 45 minutes
Makes: 12 Muffins
Calories: 189, Net Carbs: 7.5 g, Fat: 16 g, Protein: 5 g

What you need:

1 TSP of gluten-free baking powder
3/4 cup of granulated Swerve sweetener
1/2 cup of almond milk—unsweetened
1/2 cup of unsweetened cocoa powder
1/4 cup coconut oil, melted

1/3 cup of chopped stevia-sweetened dark chocolate

5 T. of softened butter

2 cups of almond flour
1 TSP of vanilla extract
1/2 TSP of salt
4 big eggs

Steps:

1. Set your stove to be the temperature of 350°F. Use baking paper or silicone cups to line a cupcake pan.
2. Using a medium bowl for mixing, thoroughly whisk almond powder, sweetener, baking powder, salt, & cocoa powder to ensure that it is blended well. Slowly blend in the coconut oil into the batter.

3. Whisk the vanilla extract, almond milk, and eggs together using a medium-sized bowl. In the bowl of dried ingredients, slowly pour out the mixture into it. Continue stirring until completely mixed.
4. Fold in the chocolate that is chopped into the batter carefully.
5. Distribute the batter into the muffin cups. Put in the heated stove for around 25 to 28 mins. or until they pass the clean toothpick test.

Egg Muffins

Total Prep & Cooking Time: 25 minutes.

Makes: 6 Servings

Calories: 168, Net Carbs: 1 g, Fat: 13 g, Protein: 12 g

What you need:

6 ounces of shredded cheese

5 ounces of chorizo or cooked bacon

12 large eggs

2 finely chopped scallions

Salt and pepper, to taste

Butter to grease muffin pan

2 T. of pesto (optional)

Steps:

1. Set the oven to preheat to the temperature of 350°F. Use butter or cooking spray to heavily grease the cupcake pan.
2. Add the chopped chorizo or bacon along with the scallions to the bottom of each cup of the cupcake pan.
3. In a medium bowl, stir the seasonings and pesto. Once mixed well, add and stir the cheese thoroughly.
4. Distribute the batter evenly to each muffin cup over the meat and scallions.
5. Bake the muffins in about 15 to 20 mins. until they turn into golden.

French Toast Muffins

Total Prep & Cooking Time: 30 minutes.

Makes: 12 Muffins

Calories: 115, Net Carbs: 1 g, Fat: 9 g, Protein: 6 g

What you need:

1 TSP of gluten-free baking powder

8 large eggs

8 ounces of cream cheese

2 TSPs of cinnamon

Steps:

1. Set the oven to heat at 400°F. Use parchment paper or silicone muffin cups to line the cupcake tray.
2. Using an electric or stand mixer, combine the cinnamon, eggs, baking powder, and cream cheese until a smooth consistency. Do not over-mix the ingredients as they will not rise properly.
3. Dispense the batter into the cups. Heat the muffins in the stove for 18 to 20 mins. until they are fluffy.
4. Serve them warm.

Pumpkin Cream Cheese Muffins

Total Prep & Cooking Time: 30 minutes.

Makes: 12 Muffins

Calories: 261, Net Carbs: 6 g, Fat: 22 g, Protein: 7 g

What you need:

4 TSPs of gluten-free baking powder

2/3 cup of granulated swerve sweetener

8 ounces of softened cream cheese

1/2 cup of coconut flour

2 TSPs of pumpkin pie spice

¾ cup of pumpkin puree

1 1/2 cups almond flour

4 large eggs

½ cup butter—softened

1 TSP of vanilla extract

½ TSP of salt

Steps:

1. Set the oven to a temperature of 350°F to preheat. Place silicone or parchment paper muffin cups into the cupcake tray.
2. Cream the sweetener & butter until it becomes fluffy and light in the big mixing bowl. Put into the mixture one egg, mixing thoroughly in between. Repeat until all eggs are combined. Add the vanilla and pumpkin puree until mixed well.

3. Stir the baking powder, almond flour, salt, coconut flour, and pumpkin spice in a medium-sized bowl, whisking to remove all lumps.
4. Combine the dry & wet ingredients into the bowl. Using a spatula made of rubber, stir it until fully mixed.
5. In the muffin cups, use a spoon to place the batter in it and then put the cream cheese in heaping tablespoons to each. Swirl the batter and cream cheese with a toothpick or butter knife for the desired look.
6. In the oven, put the muffin tray for 20 to 25 mins. or until the muffin batter (not the cream cheese!) comes out clean with a toothpick.
7. Serve at room temperature or chilled to your taste.

Raspberry Lemonade Muffins

Total Prep & Cooking Time: 45 minutes.

Makes: 8 Muffins

Calories: 255, Net Carbs: 1 g, Net Fat: 8 g, Protein: 3 g

What you need:

1 cup of blanched almond flour

1/8 TSP of vanilla flavored stevia

1 cup of frozen raspberries

1/8 TSP of gluten-free baking soda

3 big eggs

1/4 cup of grapeseed oil

1/8 TSP of salt

1 T. of lemon zest

Steps:

1. Set the stove to a temperature of 350°F. Line the muffin pan w/ 8 silicone muffin cups and/or parchment paper cups.
2. Using the food processor on high temperature, pound the baking soda, the salt, & the almond & until blended. After that, add the grapeseed oil, eggs, and lemon zest. Pulse for an additional 20 seconds.
3. Carefully stir in the frozen raspberries to the batter with a large rubber spatula.
4. Transfer evenly in the paper cups and heat for 30 mins or until all muffins become brown.
5. Cool up to 30 mins. before serving.

Chapter 5: Cookie Recipes

Chocolate Sea Salt Cookies

Total Prep & Cooking Time: 30 minutes
Makes: 12 Cookies
Calories: 149, Net Carbs: 1.6 g, Fat: 13 g, Protein: 2 g

What you need:

3/4 cup of monk fruit sweetener
1 TSP of vanilla extract
1/2 TSP of baking soda
2 cup almond flour
3/4 cup of coconut oil
2 T. of unsweetened cocoa powder
1/2 TSP of salt
1/4 TSP of cream of tartar
2 big eggs
Flaky sea salt for topping

Steps:

1. Set the temperature of the stove to 350°F. Using two cookie sheets of regular size, place 2 silicone baking mats in line or on top with the baking paper.
2. Using a bowl for mixing, you need to cream the coconut oil extract, eggs, & vanilla using the electric beater. Add the cocoa powder, monk fruit sweetener, cream of tartar, salt, & baking soda till they're mixed well.

3. Slowly add the almond flour to the dough, making sure all lumps are removed.
4. Roll the dough into balls and lightly press them 2-3 inches apart on the baking sheets. Scatter the flaky sea salt on the top of the cookies to taste.
5. Put a baking sheet one-by-one into the oven for 15 to 18 mins. and check with the toothpick test in the middle of the cookies.
6. From the stove, remove the baking sheets & put the cookies on the wire rack at least 30 mins. before serving.

Coconut Cookies

Total Prep & Cooking Time: 17 minutes

Makes: 24 Cookies

Calories: 132, Net Carbs: 1.2 g, Protein: 3 g, Net Fat: 13 g

What you need:

For the cookie dough:

1/2 cup of coconut flour

3/4 cup of monk fruit sweetener

1/2 TSP of baking soda

1/2 TSP of xanthan gum

2 TSPs of vanilla extract

2 cups of almond flour

1/2 cup of softened butter

2 large eggs

3/4 cup of unsweetened, shredded coconut

1/4 cup of softened coconut oil

1/4 TSP of salt

For the frosting:

2 T. of softened butter

1 TSP of vanilla extract

1/2 cup of monk fruit sweetener

2 T. of heavy cream

4 ounces of cream cheese

Steps:

1. Set the oven to a temperature of 350°F. Use one sheet of baking paper for a regular-sized cookie sheet.
2. Mix coconut flour, xanthan gum, and almond flour in a big bowl for mixing. Then combine the baking soda & the salt. Put it aside.
3. Using an additional large bowl, blend the eggs, coconut oil, sweetener, butter, and vanilla extract through the use of the electric blender. Slowly add ingredients which are dry that were set to the side. Once thoroughly mixed, fold in the shredded coconut into the batter.
4. Use cookie scoop or spoon to drop the dough evenly on a cookie sheet.
5. Then bake it for 12 to 15 mins., and the cookies will be brown on the edges.
6. In the meantime, using the medium-sized bowl, mix all frosting ingredients. Combine monk fruit sweetener and cream cheese until combined. Then put the vanilla extract, heavy whipping cream, & butter until the topping is thick.
7. From the oven, get the cookies & apply the frosting on the cookies with a rubber spatula after they have fully cooled.

Florentine Cookies

Total Prep & Cooking Time: 25 minutes
Makes: 8 Cookies
Calories: 275, Net Carbs: 9 g, Protein: 8 g, Net Fat: 25 g

What you need:

1/4 cup of granulated swerve sweetener
2 T. of butter
1/2 TSP of molasses
1 cup of coarsely ground almonds
1/4 cup of heavy cream
3 ounces of bar your favorite sugar-free chocolate
1 T. of gelatin

Steps:

1. Set your oven to heat to the temperature of 350°F. Using silicone mats or baking paper, line two cookie sheets.
2. Using a small-sized saucepan, mix butter, molasses, sweetener, & heavy cream on high or medium heat up to boiling for 1 minute. Turn the burner off and fold in ground almonds. Set the bowl aside for 20 mins. to cool.
3. After the pan has cooled, continue stirring the gelatin unto the mixture & put heaping tablespoons onto the prepared baking sheets. Spread the dough into thin circles.
4. Put the cookies in the oven for 10 mins. They will be cooked when the edges are brown.

5. Using a saucepan on low/medium heat, melt the chocolate making sure to stir so it will not to burn.
6. Take the cookies out of the oven and spread the base of the cookie with a thin chocolate layer with a spatula. Taking another cookie, put it on top of the chocolate.
7. Place the sandwiches in the refrigerator to cool which will make them crisper.

Nutty Cookies

Total Prep & Cooking Time: 20 minutes

Makes: 15 Cookies

Calories: 275, Net Carbs: 9 g, Protein Content: 8 g, Net Fat: 25 g

What you need:

1 cup of unsweetened and flaked coconut

1/2 cup of macadamia nuts—raw

2 T. of melted butter

1/2 cup of raw pecans

1/4 TSP of sea salt

Steps:

1. In the food processor, combine the pecans, macadamia nuts, and salt and pulsate the ingredients for 3 to 5 minutes on high until batter becomes really smooth.
2. Use a spatula made of rubber to spoon the batter to a large bowl, stirring in the coconut flakes and butter until fully combined.
3. Place parchment paper on 2 regular sized baking sheets. Use a cookie scoop or spoon and place approximately 2 TSPs of dough onto the baking sheet for each cookie.
4. Shape and flatten each cookie by hand to the desired thickness and place in the freezer for them to cool properly.
5. Take the cookies out in 1 to 2 hours after they have set.

Nutty Chocolate Chip Cookies

Total Prep & Cooking Time: 30 minutes
Makes: 16 Cookies
Calories: 177, Fat: 17 g, Protein Content: 4 g, Net Carbs: 2 g

What you need:

1/2 cup of confectioner Swerve sweetener
1/4 cup of coconut flour
1 1/4 cups of almond flour
1/2 cup of unsalted and melted butter
2 TSPs of baking powder, gluten-free
1/2 cup of macadamia nuts
1/2 cup of pistachios
1/4 cup Pyure Stevia blend
1/2 cup of **unsweetened** dark chocolate chips
1 TSP of vanilla extract
1/2 TSP of pink salt
1/2 TSP of xanthan gum (optional)
2 large eggs

Steps:

1. Set your stove to a temperature of 350°F. Using parchment paper, line the regular-sized sheet for baking or alternatively use a silicone baking mat.
2. In a small cooking pot, soften the butter on low heat.
3. Using a large bowl, you need to completely cream the eggs & pour melted butter into the bowl to mix. Put the Swerve, Pyure, & vanilla extract & mix till blended well.

4. Whisk the almond flour & coconut flour in another mixing bowl. Then pour the salt & the baking powder until completely mixed. Then put the mixture slowly & never overmix it.
5. In the dough, fold in the chocolate chips, pistachios, & macadamia nuts.
6. On a baking sheet, make small balls of dough of about 2 tablespoons and flatten them by hand.
7. Put in the heated stove for 12 to 14 mins. leaving it to become cold on a cookie sheet on the counter in approximately 5 mins.

Oatmeal Cookies

Total Prep & Cooking Time: 30 minutes

Makes: 20 Cookies

Calories: 119, Protein: 3 g, Net Carbs: 3 g, Fat: 11 g

What you need:

2 T. of oat fiber

1/2 TSP vanilla extract

1/3 cup Sukrin Gold (used as a substitute for brown sugar)

1/4 TSP of baking soda

1 1/2 cups of sliced almonds

A cup of almond flour

1/4 TSP of salt

1 large egg

3/4 TSP of cinnamon

2 TSP of beef gelatin

4 ounces of unsalted and softened butter

Steps:

1. Set the stove to heat at 350°F. Use silicone baking mats or two parchment paper lined regular sized cookie sheets.
2. Using the food processor, pour sliced almonds inside & pulse on low speed until they are chunky.
3. Mix the brown sugar, vanilla, and butter extract until light into the medium-sized mixing bowl.
4. Using a large bowl, add the baking soda, almond flour, cinnamon, oat fiber, beef gelatin, and salt and then continue the stir until mixed well.

5. Beat in the egg until the dough is thoroughly mixed. Fold in the chopped almonds unto the dough.
6. Then you need to use a cookie scoop, so you can drop the dough approximately 2 inches from each other onto the cookie sheet.
7. Heat the cookies for 8 minutes and remove. Gently knock the baking sheet on the counter to make the cookies flatten. Put the pan back in the stove for 6 additional minutes.
8. Leave for 5 minutes on a cooling rack and serve once cooled.

Tricks and Tips:

- If you prefer a wider and flatter cookie, use only 1 cup of sliced almonds in this recipe. Using the recommended 1 1/2 cups of sliced almonds will give you a smaller cookie that is thicker.
- When measuring out the oat fiber and almond flour, be sure not to pack the ingredients in the measuring cups. This will result in the cookies being too dry as there will be too much of the ingredient included in the recipe.

Oreo Cookies

Total Prep & Cooking Time: 1 hour 25 minutes

Makes: 18 Cookies

Calories: 112, Net Carbs: 2 g, Protein Content: 1 g, Net Fat: 12 g

What you need:

For the cookie dough:

1/4 cup of granulated Swerve sweetener

2 cups of almond flour

1/2 cup of unsalted & softened butter

1/3 cup of unsweetened cocoa powder

1 TSP of fine sea salt

For the Filling:

1 cup of confectioner Swerve sweetener

1/2 cup of unsalted butter softened

Steps:

1. Set the stove to heat at the temperature of 350°F. Using baking paper, line a regular sized cookie sheet. Prepare an additional piece of parchment paper and set to the side.
2. Mix the cocoa powder, sweetener, almond flour, & salt inside the big mixing bowl. Using the fork, whisk to ensure there are no dry patches or lumps. Add in the butter until the consistency of the batter is smooth.
3. On the additional piece of baking paper, roll the dough into a

log 1 1/2 inches thick.
4. Cool the dough in the fridge for approximately 1 hour until firm.
5. While the dough is firming up, beat the butter and powdered sweetener for the filling with an electric beater until incorporated.
6. Take the dough out and cut the log with a thin, sharp knife into slices about 1/4 inches thick.
7. Spacing approximately 2 inches apart, put cookies unto the piece of a cookie sheet.
8. And then, you need to bake it for 15 to 12 mins. and remove. Put the cookie baking sheet on the counter at least 10 mins. for it to cool. Then move the cookies with a spatula to a wire rack. This will keep the cookies from crumbling.
9. On a cookie, spread a small amount of filling. Take another cookie on the top. Repeat & enjoy!

Tricks and Tips:

- Dutched cocoa is highly recommended for this recipe is it contains higher levels of fat and adds more flavor to the cookies. It also neutralizes acidity as it is processed with alkali.
- The coloring of the cookies will have the classic Oreo look as they will be darker compared to regular cocoa powder, and the dutched cocoa will give the cookies a more intense chocolate flavor.

Vanilla Crescent Cookies

Total Prep & Cooking Time: 30 minutes

Makes: 14 Cookies

Calories: 132, Net Carbs: 1.2 g, Protein Content: 3 g, Net Fat: 13 g

What you need:

For the cookie dough:

4 T. of ground almonds
2 1/2 T. of granulated sweetener
1/2 cup of finely ground almond flour
1/2 TSP of sugar-free vanilla extract
1/4 cup of softened butter
1 vanilla of bean pod

For the topping:

2 T. of powdered sweetener

Steps:

1. Set your oven to a temperature of 350°F. Use parchment paper or a silicone mat to line a regular sized cookie sheet.
2. Using an electric beater, cream the sweetener & the butter in the big bowl till combined.
3. Open now the vanilla's pod & get the seeds out and discard. Put the remaining pod in the mixing bowl. Add the ground almonds, almond flour, and vanilla extract into the mixing bowl until it is a slightly crumbly consistency.

4. Scoop approximately 1 T. of dough to form into half-moon shapes and space them one to two inches away from the prepared baking cookie sheet.
5. Next, heat the cookie tray for 10 minutes and set them out to cool for 30 minutes on the tray.
6. When they are cooled, roll the cookies in the confectioner sweetener until they are covered entirely.

Chapter 6: Bun and Bagel Recipes

Bun Recipes

Dinner Rolls

Total Prep & Cooking Time: 1 hour 10 minutes
Makes: 12 Rolls
Calories: 75, Net Carbs: 2 g, Protein Content: 3 g, Net Fat: 5 g

What you need:

2 T. of psyllium husk powder

8 T. of coconut flour

3 TSPs of gluten-free baking powder

1 medium of finely grated zucchini

2 T. of apple cider vinegar

2 T. of avocado oil

1 T. of dried basil

4 large eggs

1/4 cup of water

1/2 TSP of salt

Method:

1. Set the stove to 350°F to preheat. Put a heavy grease on the baking pan using butter and set it aside.
2. Mix the baking powder, coconut flour, psyllium husk powder, dried basil, and salt into a big mixing bowl, and mix it thoroughly.

3. In the medium-sized mixing bowl, you need to thoroughly stir the eggs, apple cider vinegar, avocado oil, & water. Add in the shredded zucchini to the batter.
4. Put the mixture slowly into the bowl of dry ingredient and combine them using an electric mixer to mix completely.
5. Take the dough and create the size and shape rolls you prefer by hand (dinner or round rolls) and place on the prepared sheet pan.
6. Brush the avocado oil on unbaked bread & put inside an oven for 40 to 45 mins. & serve warm.

Hawaiian Sweet Rolls

Total Prep & Cooking Time: 30 minutes

Makes: 10 Rolls

Calories: 189, Net Carbs: 6.2 g, Protein: 16 g, Fat: 12 g

What you need:

2 TSP of gluten-free baking powder

3 ounces of cream cheese

1 1/2 cups of almond flour

6 drops of pineapple oil

2 large eggs

3/4 cup of confectioner Swerve sweetener

1 TSP of fresh ginger paste

Steps:

1. Measure all ingredients ahead of time to be prepared for when the mozzarella cheese melts, as the ingredients will need to be combined quickly. There will be no time to measure while preparing this dish.
2. Set the stove to heat at 425°F. Liberally grease a regular sized sheet pan.
3. Stir together the baking powder, Swerve sweetener, and almond flour using a medium bowl until combined well.
4. Use a double boiler to melt the cream cheese and mozzarella and pour into the bowl, stirring until incorporated.
5. Add the fresh ginger paste, pineapple oil and eggs to the mixture and blend until the dough has a sticky texture.
6. Using the baking paper or a non-stick mat, knead the dough

until it becomes less sticky. It will have some tacky quality when complete.

7. Slice into ten pieces the bread dough and create a ball by rolling by hand.
8. Place all the dough balls so they are all touching into the lined sheet pan.
9. Heat the rolls for 15 to 20 mins. in the oven. The rolls will have a golden crust when complete.
10. Using a knife, separate the lines in the bread before pulling the rolls out. The bottom of the rolls will have a golden-brown crust as well.

Mini Buns

Total Prep & Cooking Time: 15 minutes

Makes: 6 Servings

Calories: 357, Net Carbs: 9 g, Protein: 13 g, Fat: 31 g

What you need:

1/4 cup of melted butter

1 T. of dried herbs of your preference i.e. oregano, rosemary, thyme, or dill

1 cup almond flour—blanched

2 T. of sesame seeds

4 large eggs

1/2 TSP of pink salt

Finely grated Parmesan cheese (optional)

Steps:

1. Set your oven to a temperature of 425°F. Use butter to heavily grease a small loaf pan or line with baking paper.
2. On a high temperature, thoroughly blend butter, eggs, the almond flour, herb(s) of your preference, and sesame seeds using a food processor. Continue this until it becomes a smooth consistency.
3. Use a spatula made of rubber or spoon to distribute evenly the dough unto the prepared muffin cups.
4. If you prefer, add parmesan cheese on top of the buns before baking.
5. Bake it for 10 to 12 mins. and leave it in the pan for at least 5 mins. To the complete cooling process, transfer to a wire rack.

Sesame Buns

Total Prep & Cooking Time: 15 minutes
Makes: 12 Buns
Calories: 133, Net Carbs: 4 g, Fat: 7 g, Protein: 7 g

What you need:

1/2 cup of psyllium powder
8 egg whites
1 cup of coconut flour
1 T. of sea salt
1 cup of sesame seeds
1 T. baking powder—gluten-free
1 cup of hot water
1/2 cup of pumpkin seeds

Steps:

1. Set your oven to 350°F to make sure it is preheated. Use the sheet of "parchment paper" or use a non-stick mat to line the baking sheet.
2. Combine the baking powder, psyllium powder, 1/2 cup of the sesame seeds, coconut flour, pumpkin seeds, and sea salt in a big bowl until thoroughly mixed.
3. In a blender, cream the egg whites until light and stir into the dry ingredient bowl.
4. Slowly mix the hot water to the batter and stir for approximately 1 minute until the dough becomes smoother. It will still have a crumbly consistency when complete. Let the dough stand for 5 minutes before continuing.

5. Form the small buns by hand and place them on a plate to pour the remaining sesame seeds over them. On the prepared cookie sheet, transfer the buns once complete.
6. Bake it for 45 to 50 mins. and turn the oven off when they have a golden crust. Leave them in the oven to cool for them to become crispier if you prefer.

Tricks and Tips:

- When choosing the coconut flour, you will use in this recipe, be sure to buy the lightest and finest flour that is available. If a rougher version of coconut flour is used, this will result in the bread being less fluffy and denser. Look in Chapter 3 for coconut flours which will be the proper variety for this particular recipe.
- There should be no dry patches present in the dough to ensure the bun will properly stick together as you shape the buns. If there are still dry patches present after kneading, add hot water in small amounts and mix to eliminate.

Bagel Recipes

Blueberry Cheesecake Bagels

Total Prep & Cooking Time: 40 minutes
Makes: 12 Bagels
Calories: 68, Net Carbs: 3.3 g, Protein Content: 4 g, Net Fat: 5 g

What you need:

3/4 cup of almond flour
3/4 cup of nut flour
2 T of granulated Swerve sweetener
1 T. of baking powder—gluten-free
1 large egg (needed for egg wash)
1/2 cup of blueberries
2 ounces of cream cheese
2 large eggs
2 1/2 cups of shredded mozzarella cheese

Steps:

1. Set your oven to heat at 400°F. Cover a regular sized cookie sheet with baking paper or use a heavily greased donut tray.
2. Use a double boiler to melt the cream cheese and mozzarella cheese together. Once melted, add 2 eggs and thoroughly beat.
3. Combine half of the Swerve (1 T.), baking powder, nut flour, & almond flour in the big bowl. Mix them thoroughly. Pour into the melted cheese and start kneading the dough by hand.
4. Carefully stir in the fresh blueberries with a rubber spatula and then split the dough into 8 equal balls.

5. On parchment paper or silicone mat, roll the individual balls into logs to your preferred thickness of bagel. Connect the two ends together to create a circle.
6. Place the bagels into the donut tray or cookie sheet. Using the egg wash, brush each bagel with a pastry brush and sprinkle the Swerve on top of them.
7. Put the tray on the stove and heat it for 10 to 14 mins.
8. Transfer it to the cooling rack for about 15 mins. and serve.

Cheese Bagels

Total Prep & Cooking Time: 40 minutes

Makes: 6 Bagels

Calories: 356, Net Carbs: 6 g, Fat: 28 g, Protein: 23 g

What you need:

3 T. of coconut flour

1 TSP of baking soda

2 ounces of cream cheese

2 1/2 cups of shredded mozzarella

1 1/2 cups of almond flour

2 TSPs of cream of tartar

2 large eggs

2 TSPs of sesame seeds

1 large egg for egg wash

Steps:

1. Set the oven to the temperature of 400°F to heat. Cover a regular sized cookie sheet with baking paper or use a heavily greased donut tray.
2. Whisk the almond flour and coconut flour in the big bowl. Then put the tartar cream & the baking soda & continue whisking to remove all lumps.
3. Use a double boiler to melt the cream cheese and mozzarella cheese together on medium/high heat.
4. Cream 1 egg until beaten in a small bowl and repeat for the additional egg. Combine slowly to the dry ingredient bowl and mix until together. Then add the melted cheese to the flour

mixture and work the dough together by kneading.
5. Split the dough into 6 individual balls. Using the sheet of baking paper, you need to roll each dough ball into logs to your preferred thickness of bagel. Connect the two ends of the dough together.
6. Place the bagels on the lined cookie sheet or donut tray. Using the egg wash, brush each bagel with a pastry brush and dust the sesame seeds on top of them.
7. Put in the oven for 15 to 17 mins. They will have a golden texture when complete.
8. Transfer for 30 mins. to a cooling rack before serving.

Jalapeno Bagels

Total Prep & Cooking Time: 40 minutes

Makes: 6 Bagels

Calories: 273, Net Carbs: 6 g, Protein: 16 g, Fat: 22 g

What you need:

1 TSP of baking powder

2 cups of grated mozzarella cheese

2 ounces of cream cheese

1 cup of almond flour

1 ounce of grated cheddar cheese

2 large eggs

3 medium jalapeno peppers

Steps:

1. Set the oven to heat at 400°F. Use a heavily greased donut tray or parchment paper on a regular sized cookie sheet.
2. Cut open the jalapeno peppers and remove the seeds. Cut the jalapeno peppers into thin slices and set to the side.
3. Whisk the flour of the almond & the baking powder inside the big bowl in order to remove any and all lumps.
4. Use the double boiler on high or medium heat in order to melt the cream cheese and mozzarella cheese. Once melted, add to the dry ingredient bowl and thoroughly knead the dough.
5. Divide the dough into individual balls. Roll the individual balls into logs on parchment paper to your preferred size of the bagel. Connect the two ends together to finish the bagels.
6. Move the bagels on the cookie sheet. Put the sliced jalapeno

peppers on each bagel and sprinkle the cheddar cheese on the bagels.
7. Heat in the stove for 25 to 30 mins. Serve hot for the best taste.

Pizza Bagel Bites

Total Prep & Cooking Time: 25 minutes

Makes: 10 Bagels

Calories: 110, Net Carbs: 5 g, Fat: 15 g, Protein: 14 g

What you need:

For the bagel dough:

2 T. of almond flour, separate

3/4 cups of almond flour

1 ounce of cream cheese

5 cups of shredded mozzarella cheese

2 TSP of gluten-free baking powder

1 large egg

1 large egg for egg wash

For bagel topping:

3 cups of minced pepperoni

1/1/3 cups of low-sugar pizza sauce

1/3 cup of shredded mozzarella cheese

Steps:

1. Set the oven temperature to 400°F. Place parchment paper on 2 regular sized baking sheets or use 2 heavily greased donut trays.
2. Using a fork, whisk thoroughly the almond flour & the baking powder inside the big bowl, ensuring that no more lumps are

there. Beat the egg to the mixture to combine thoroughly.
3. Use a double boiler to melt the cream cheese and mozzarella cheese together. Once melted, add to the dry ingredients to create the bread dough.
4. Split into individual balls. Roll the balls into logs on parchment paper to your preferred thickness of bagel. Creating a circle, connect the two ends of the dough together.
5. Place the bagels on the prepared donut tray or cookie sheet. Apply the egg wash with a pastry brush to the tops of the bagels and place one tray at a time in the stove for 5 minutes until they are puffy and golden.
6. Cut the bagels in half and top with the pizza sauce, mozzarella cheese and pepperoni and put the tray back in to bake for an additional 3 minutes for the toppings to heat. Serve hot and enjoy!

Chapter 7: Bread Loaf Recipes

Blueberry Bread Loaf

Total Prep & Cooking Time: 30 minutes
Makes: 12 Slices
Calories: 155, Net Carbs: 4 g, Fat: 13 g, Protein: 3 g

What you need:

For the bread dough:

10 T. of coconut flour

9 T. of melted butter

2/3 cup of granulated Swerve sweetener

1 1/2 TSP of gluten-free baking powder

2 T. of heavy whipping cream

1 1/2 TSPs of vanilla extract

1/2 TSP of cinnamon

2 T. of sour cream

6 large eggs

1/2 TSP of salt

3/4 cup of blueberries

For the topping:

1 T. of heavy whipping cream

2 T. of confectioner Swerve sweetener

1 TSP of melted butter

1/8 TSP of vanilla extract

1/4 TSP of lemon zest

Steps:

1. Set your oven to heat at 350°F. Use a silicone bread pan or baking paper to line a regular sized loaf pan.
2. In a big mixing bowl, thoroughly mix the heavy whipping cream, granulated Srweve, eggs, and baking powder. Once combined, add the sour cream, cinnamon, salt, vanilla extract and butter. Lastly, add the coconut flour to the batter.
3. Pour a layer about 1/2 inch of dough into the bread pan. Place 1/4 cup of blueberries on top of the dough. Keep repeating until the dough and blueberry layers are complete.
4. For 65 to 75 mins, bake it inside the oven. Use any utensil to push into the middle of the bread loaf to ensure properly baked.
5. While the bread is in the stove, use a small bowl to beat the confectioner Swerve, lemon zest, heavy whipping cream, butter, and vanilla extract. Mix until creamy.
6. On a heatproof surface, move the pan after the bread loaf is cooked to let it cool for five mins. Drizzle the icing topping on the bread.
7. Allow to fully cool before slicing and serve.

Cauliflower Bread Loaf

Total Prep & Cooking Time: 1 hour 10 minutes
Makes: 10 Slices
Calories: 155, Net Carbs: 4 g, Fat: 13 g, Protein: 3 g

What you need:

For the bread dough:

1 1/4 cups of almond flour
3 cups of riced cauliflower
1 T. of gluten-free baking powder
6 T. of olive oil
6 large eggs, separated
1 TSP salt

Optional flavoring ingredients:

Dried or fresh herbs such as rosemary, oregano and/or thyme
Shredded parmesan or cheddar cheese
Garlic powder or minced garlic

Steps:

1. Set the temperature of the oven to heat at 350°F. Use a non-stick bread pan or line a regular sized loaf pan with baking paper.
2. Place cauliflower into the small pot to steam until it becomes tender. Place it to the side.
3. In a food processor set on high, cream the whites of the eggs

for 4 minutes. Set to the side.
4. In a large-sized bowl, put the almond flour & egg yolks, whisking till combined thoroughly. Next, add the baking powder, oil & salt and stir until smooth.
5. Place the cooled cauliflower in a paper towel or a tea towel and turn clockwise to remove any excess fluid.
6. Stir in the dried cauliflower and mix well. Add the optional flavoring ingredients if you choose to add variety.
7. In small amounts, fold the egg white mixture to the mixture until fluffy. Be sure not to mix too thoroughly so that the egg whites remain airy and fluffy, ensuring the bread will properly rise.
8. Transfer the dough into the bread loaf pan.
9. Place it into an oven for 45 mins. Use the knife test to make sure the loaf is baked through.
10. Allow the bread loaf to completely cool before slicing and serving.

Tricks and Tips:

- This bread is quite similar in appearance to a regular white loaf bread except that it does not rise as high. This is correct for the cauliflower bread loaf, so do not fret if it appears to have fallen.
- Ensure the cauliflower is properly riced (see Chapter 1 for instructions) so that it looks more like grainy crumb consistency compared to how it would appear for a cauliflower rice dish.

Cheese and Bacon Bread Loaf

Total Prep & Cooking Time: 1 hour

Makes: 10 Slices

Calories: 292, Net Carbs: 4 g, Protein Content: 3 g, Net Fat: 13 g

What you need:

1/3 of cup sour cream

4 T of melted butter

1 1/2 cups of almond flour

1 cup of grated cheese of your preference

1 T. of gluten-free baking powder

2 large eggs

200 g of bacon

Steps:

1. Set your oven to a temperature of 300°F. Line the loaf pan with baking paper or you can also use a silicone-based bread pan.
2. Cut & dice the bacon & use a large frying pan to cook until crispy.
3. In the small-sized cooking pan, you need to heat the butter & set aside for it to cool down.
4. Use a large-sized bowl in mixing the baking powder and almond flour with a fork to ensure all lumps are removed.
5. Using an electric beater, cream the sour cream and eggs into the flour mix. Add to the mixed dry ingredient bowl along with the cooled butter and combine well.
6. Fold in the grated cheese and cooked bacon into the dough.

7. Empty the dough into the bread loaf pan. If you want the bread to be extra cheesy, sprinkle the top with extra cheese at this time.
8. Bake if for at least 45 to 50 mins. Using a utensil, test the middle of the bread loaf.
9. Keep the bread on the counter to completely cool or in the refrigerator before slicing and serving.

Tricks and Tips:

- Cooling the cheese and bacon bread loaf in the refrigerator instead of on the counter will ensure that the loaf will not crumble while slicing. This will also make the bread denser, making it easier to cut.
- If you prefer the bread warm, you can place it back in the oven to heat it up or the microwave before putting the desired toppings on the bread slice. It is not recommended to put the bread slices in a toaster.

Hearty Seeded Bread Loaf

Total Prep & Cooking Time: 1 hour 10 minutes
Makes: 16 Slices
Calories: 172, Net Carbs: 2 g, Protein Content: 7 g, Net Fat: 6 g

What you need:

1 1/2 cups pumpkin seeds—raw and shelled

1/2 cup of whole psyllium husks

1/2 cup of flax seeds

1/2 cup of chia seeds

1 1/2 cups of warm water

1 TSP of pink salt

1 cup of raw sunflower seeds

1 T. of maple syrup

3 T. of melted coconut oil

Steps:

1. Set your oven to a temperature of 350°F. Use a silicone bread pan or use parchment paper to line a regular sized loaf pan.
2. Chop one cup of pumpkin seeds through using the food processor until finely chopped. The consistency of should be of medium-coarse flour.
3. In a big bowl, pour in the remaining pumpkin seeds (1/2 cup), pumpkin seed flour, sunflower seeds, psyllium husks, chia seed, flax seeds, and salt.
4. Pour the warm water, maple syrup, & melted coconut oil into a mixing bowl & continue stirring until the batter becomes thick.

5. Pack the batter by hand into the lined bread loaf pan.
6. Bake the loaf for 45 minutes and remove the pan. On a sheet of baking paper put the bread loaf, turned over on the top and remove the bread pan from the loaf of bread.
7. Return the bread to the oven to continue cooking for approximately 15 more minutes.
8. Allow the bread loaf to completely cool before slicing and serving.

Pumpkin Bread Loaf

Total Prep & Cooking Time: 1 hour

Makes: 10 Slices

Calories: 165, Net Carbs: 6 g, Protein Content: 5 g, Net Fat: 14 g

What you need:

1/2 cup of coconut flour

1 1/2 cups of almond flour

4 TSPs of gluten-free baking powder

1/2 cup of softened butter

1 TSP of cinnamon

4 large eggs

2/3 cup of granulated Swerve sweetener

3/4 cup of pumpkin puree

1/2 TSP of nutmeg

1/4 TSP of ginger

1/8 TSP of cloves

1 TSP of vanilla extract

1/2 TSP of salt

Steps:

1. The oven needs to be set to 350°F to heat. Cover a bread loaf pan with baking paper or use a silicone bread pan.
2. Mix the butter & sweetener in a big bowl using an electric beater until light.
3. Put 1 egg into the batter and whisk well. Repeat for all the eggs to ensure the batter is well mixed.
4. Combine the vanilla extract and pumpkin puree into the

batter, mixing thoroughly.
5. Mix the ingredients like the almond & coconut flour, & the baking powder into the separate big mixing bowl to remove all lumps. Then add the nutmeg, cinnamon, cloves, ginger, and salt, whisking to remove any additional lumps.
6. Combine the puree to the bowl of dry ingredients & mix thoroughly the batter well.
7. Transfer the completed dough into the lined bread loaf pan.
8. Heat in the stove for 45 to 50 mins. Test with a utensil until it comes out without batter.
9. To make sure it will not crumble, the bread loaf needs to be cooled completely.

Tricks and Tips:

- If pumpkin spice is not available, it is quite easy to make your own homemade recipe. You will need the following ingredients:

    o 1 1/2 TSP of ground cinnamon
    o 1/2 TSP of ground nutmeg
    o 1/2 TSP of ground ginger
    o 1/4 TSP of ground cloves
    o 1/4 TSP of ground allspice

Simply whisk all spices together using a small bowl and this will make 1 T. worth of spice. The left-over pumpkin spice can be easily stored in an airtight dish afterwards.

- You can also use this pumpkin recipe to make muffins instead of the bread loaf. Pour the batter into 12 silicone muffin liners or parchment lined muffin tray. The oven will be pre-heated to the proper temperature of 350°F, but the cooking time will diminish to 25 minutes.
- There are several flavoring varieties you can incorporate into this recipe. If you would like to add chopped pecans or walnuts, add 1/2 cup to the batter before pouring into the bread loaf pan.
- For the sweet tooth, you can add 1/2 cup of low-carb chocolate chips to the dough before placing in the loaf pan.
- For an even sweeter variety, you can top the pumpkin bread loaf with cream cheese frosting. This is will require the following ingredients:
  - 1/2 cup of Swerve, confectioner powder
  - 4 ounces of cream cheese, softened
  - 2 ounces of butter, softened
  - 1 TSP of vanilla extract
  - 1/8 TSP of salt

Combine with an electric beater the Swerve sweetener, salt, butter, vanilla extract, and creamed cheese. Then spread on top after the pumpkin bread has properly cooled. Slice and Enjoy!

Quick Low-Carb Bread Loaf

Total Prep & Cooking Time: 45 minutes

Makes: 16 Slices

Calories: 174, Net Carbs: 5 g, Protein Content: 5 g, Net Fat: 15 g

What you need:

2/3 cup coconut flour

1/2 cup butter—melted

3 T. coconut oil—melted

1 1/3 cups almond flour

1/2 TSP xanthan gum (optional)

1 TSP gluten-free baking powder

6 large eggs

1/2 TSP of salt

Steps:

1. The oven needs to be preheated to heat at 350°F. With baking paper, cover the bread loaf pan or use a silicone-based bread pan.
2. Using a food processor, beat the eggs until creamy.
3. Add in the almond flour and the coconut flour mixing them for 1 minute. Next, add the coconut oil, xanthan gum, butter, baking powder, and salt and mix them till the dough turns thick.
4. Put the completed dough into the prepared line of bread loaf pan.

5. Place in the stove for 40 to 45 mins. Using a knife, test to make sure the bread loaf is fully baked.
6. Slice the bread loaf after it has cooled completely before serving.

Savory Bread Loaf

Total Prep & Cooking Time: 1 hour

Makes: 12 Slices

Calories: 202, Net Carbs: 5 g, Protein Content: 6 g, Net Fat: 20 g

What you need:

1/4 cup of coconut flour

8 large eggs

8 ounces of cream cheese

2 1/2 cups almond flour

1/2 cup of butter

1 TSP of rosemary

1 1/2 TSPs baking powder—gluten-free

1 TSP of sage

2 T. of parsley

Steps:

1. Preheat your oven to be heated at 350°F. Using a silicone bread pan or parchment paper on a regular sized loaf pan.
2. Combine the butter, rosemary, parsley, sage, and sour cream in a regular mixing bowl until fluffy and mixed thoroughly.
3. In the mixture, whisk each egg & repeat until all eggs are mixed into the mixture and are smooth.
4. Add the coconut & almond flour & the baking powder & combine them thoroughly resulting in a thick dough.
5. In the lined bread loaf pan, pour the completed dough.

6. Heat the bread loaf in the stove for about 50 to 55 mins. Using a knife, check the middle to ensure baked properly.
7. Slice the bread loaf after it has cooled completely before serving.

Chapter 8: Pizza Crust and Breadstick Recipes

Pizza Crust Recipes

Coconut Flour Pizza Crust

Total Prep & Cooking Time: 35 minutes
Makes: 2 Crusts
Calories: 398, Net Carbs: 14 g, Protein: 14 g, Fat: 32 g

What you need:

1/4 cup of melted coconut oil

3 large eggs

1/4 cup of coconut flour

1 clove

1/4 TSP of pink salt

1 TSP baking powder—gluten-free

1 TSP of oregano (optional)

Steps:

1. Make sure the oven is set to 350°F. On a pizza sheet, or you can also use a stone pizza pan, lay a sheet of baking paper. Place an additional piece of parchment paper to the side.
2. Mix the pink salt, coconut flour, clove, baking powder, & oregano unto the medium-sized bowl and then thoroughly whisk ensuring that it is mixed well.
3. In another medium mixing bowl, whip the coconut oil and eggs together thoroughly.

4. Slowly combine with the dry ingredients and incorporate until the dough is thick.
5. Transfer the dough to the additional piece of baking paper.
6. Roll to flatten and shape the dough between 1/2 and 3/4 inches thick. Poke the bubbles in the finished product with a fork.
7. Transfer the dough on the prepared pizza plate or stone and bake it for at least 20 mins. Make sure the crust should be a golden-brown color.
8. Remove the pizza crust and complete with your favorite pizza toppings.
9. Place the pizza back into the oven for 2 to 3 minutes to heat the toppings.

Fathead Pizza Crust

Total Preparation & Cooking Time: 35 minutes

Makes: 8 Servings

Calories: 102, Net Carbs: 1.3 g, Fat: 32 g, Protein: 14 g

What you need:

2 T. of cream cheese

1 large egg

1 1/2 cups of shredded mozzarella cheese

3/4 cup of almond flour

1/8 TSP of salt

Steps:

1. Set the stove to 350°F to heat. Use a stone pizza pan or line a pizza sheet with baking paper. Place a sheet of parchment paper to the side.
2. Using a big microwave-safe bowl, add the mozzarella & cream cheeses & almond flour. Set the microwave to high and place the bowl inside. Leave for 50 to 60 seconds and remove. Stir and then put back into the microwave for an additional 30 sec.
3. Put the salt and egg to the bowl, making sure not to overmix.
4. Roll to flatten and shape the dough on parchment paper to the desired thickness. Poke the bubbles in the crust with a fork.
5. Place the dough on the prepared pizza pan or stone and bake for 12 to 17 minutes. The crust should be firm and golden.
6. Remove the pizza crust and finish with your favorite toppings.
7. Place the pizza back into the oven for 2 to 3 minutes to heat the toppings.

Zero Carb Pizza Crust

Total Prep & Cooking Time: 45 minutes

Makes: 1 Crust

Calories: 297, Net Carbs: 0 g, Protein: 30 g, Fat: 21 g

What you need:

1 lb. of ground chicken

1/4 TSP of pepper

1 T. of Italian seasoning

1/2 cup of parmesan cheese

Olive oil (optional)

1/2 cup of shredded cheddar cheese

Steps:

1. Make sure you stove is set to the temperature of 425°F. Put a sheet of baking paper on a pizza sheet or use a pizza stone. Place an additional piece of parchment paper to the side.
2. In a big bowl, combine ground chicken, cheddar cheese, Italian seasoning, salt, pepper, and parmesan cheese. Incorporate the ingredients until thick.
3. On parchment paper, roll the dough to shape and flatten to the desired thickness. Use a fork to poke any bubbles.
4. Place the dough on the prepared pizza pan or stone and bake it for at least 12 to 17 mins.
5. Remove the crust of the pizza and finish with your favorite pizza toppings. If you prefer, brush the pizza crust with olive oil after removing from the oven for additional flavor and fat content.

6. For 10 to 12 mins., again, put the pizza inside the oven for the toppings to heat.

Tricks and Tips:

- This recipe is ideal if you have an allergic reaction to flours or eggs as these are not included in the ingredients. This method can also be used for other bread recipes and adds more flavor to your dishes as well.
- The above recipe cooking time will give you a crispier crust. If you prefer something of a softer texture, simply reduce the amount of time the crust is in the oven by 5 to 7 minutes.
- For further variety, you can add spices to the crust depending on the style of pizza you are making. You could add garlic, crushed red pepper or experiment with different seasonings. The spices would need to be added with the rest of the dry ingredients before rolling the dough flat.

Breadstick Recipes

Cauliflower Breadsticks

Total Prep & Cooking Time: 25 minutes
Makes: 8 Breadsticks
Calories: 165, Net Carbs: 5 g, Protein: 13 g, Fat: 10 g

What you need:

For breadstick dough:

2 cups of riced cauliflower
1 cup mozzarella—shredded
1 TSP of Italian seasoning
2 large eggs
1/2 TSP of ground pepper
1/2 TSP of salt
1/2 TSP of granulated garlic

For the topping:

1/4 cup parmesan cheese

Steps:

1. First, set the oven to the temperature of 350°F. Liberally grease a standard-sized baking sheet using butter or simply use a baking mat that's non-stick.
2. Using a food processor, beat the eggs until mixed thoroughly.
3. Combine the prepared rice cauliflower, mozzarella cheese,

Italian seasoning, pepper, garlic, and salt and blend on low speed.
4. Pour the dough into the prepared cookie sheet and pat the dough down to make sure it is a uniform 1/4 inch-thick across the whole pan.
5. Bake the breadsticks for 30 minutes and dust the breadsticks with the parmesan cheese.
6. Put the breadsticks on the broil setting for 2 to 3 minutes so the cheese will melt.
7. Remove the bread from the pan and slice into individual breadsticks.

Tricks and tips:

- Look in Chapter 3 under Time-Saving Tips to see how to properly prepare the riced cauliflower to ensure the best results for your breadsticks.

Cheese Breadsticks

Total Prep & Cooking Time: 1 hour

Makes: 4 Breadsticks

Calories: 314, Net Carbs: 3.6 g, Protein: 18 g, Fat: 25 g

What you need:

2 TSPs baking powder—gluten-free
1 large egg
2 ounces of cream cheese
1 1/2 cups of shredded mozzarella cheese
¼ TSP of garlic powder
1/3 cup of almond flour

Steps:

1. The oven needs to be preheated to 425°F. Use a silicone baking mat or liberally grease a standard sized baking sheet with butter. You will also need parchment paper set to the side.
2. Use a double boiler to melt the cream cheese and half (3/4 cup) of the mozzarella cheese together.
3. Mix the egg and almond flour in a big bowl until mixed well. Then, put baking powder & garlic powder till well completely.
4. Slowly pour in the melted cheese and combine thoroughly.
5. Form the dough roundly and then wrap the dough with parchment paper, then put it in the refrigerator for at least 30 mins. to chill.
6. Dust a cutting board with a handful of almond flour and roll four pieces of dough into a log shape about 6 inches long.

7. Place each breadstick on the cookie sheet and dust with the remainder of the mozzarella cheese.
8. After that, bake it for 10 to 12 mins. & enjoy warm!

Garlic Breadsticks

Total Prep & Cooking Time: 30 minutes

Makes: 4 Breadsticks

Calories: 237, Net Carbs: 2.6 g, Protein: 12.8 g, Fat: 18.8 g

What you need:

1/2 cup of finely ground almond flour

1 cup of shredded mozzarella

1 T. of melted butter

1 TSP of gluten-free baking powder

1 T. of grated parmesan cheese

2 T. cream cheese

1 clove of minced garlic

1 large egg

1 T. of garlic powder

1 T. of chopped fresh parsley

Salt to taste

Steps:

1. Set your oven to heat at 400°F. Use a silicone baking mat or cover a standard sized cooking sheet with baking paper.
2. Use a double boiler to melt the cream cheese and mozzarella cheese on medium/high heat, ensuring it is smooth.
3. Combine the egg & almond flour in the big mixing bowl until mixed thoroughly. Then incorporate the baking & garlic powders unto the mixture.
4. Carefully pour in the melted cheese until mixed well. Roll & shape the dough like ovals with a thickness of 1 1/4 inches and

put it on a piece of baking sheet.
5. Whisk the parsley, garlic, parmesan cheese, and butter in a mixing bowl. Once completely mixed, use a brush the breadsticks with the seasonings.
6. Heat in the stove for 15 to 17 minutes and enjoy hot!

Italian Breadsticks

Total Prep & Cooking Time: 30 minutes

Makes: 6 Breadsticks

Calories: 238, Net Carbs: 2.8 g, Fat: 19 g, Protein: 13 g

What you need:

1 T. of pulverized psyllium husk

3/4 cup of almond flour

1 T. of flaxseed meal

3 T. of cream cheese

1 TSP baking powder—gluten-free

2 cups mozzarella cheese—shredded

2 medium eggs

1 TSP of pepper

2 TSPs of Italian seasoning

1 TSP of salt

Steps:

1. Make sure that the oven is set to heat at 400°F. Use a silicone baking mat or cover a standard sized baking sheet with baking paper.
2. Place 2 pieces of parchment paper to the side or you can use aluminum foil instead.
3. On medium heat, use a double boiler to melt the mozzarella cheese completely.
4. Meanwhile, in another bowl, combine the eggs and cream cheese until mixed thoroughly. Set to the side.
5. Whisk the psyllium husk & baking powders & almond flour

into the large-sized bowl together, removing any lumps.
6. Add in the mixture of cheese to the bowl of dry ingredient and mix thoroughly. Next, add the melted mozzarella cheese to the batter.
7. Knead the dough by hand until thick.
8. Use a rolling pin to press the dough flat on parchment paper, keeping an even thickness throughout.
9. Transfer the flattened dough to a piece of aluminum foil or the additional piece of parchment paper to cut into strips with a pizza cutter.
10. Sprinkle the salt, Italian seasoning and pepper on each breadstick.
11. Put it on a piece of cookie sheet & then you need to bake it for 13-15 mins. and serve warm.

Rosemary Sea Salt Breadsticks

Total Prep & Cooking Time: 30 minutes

Makes: 30 Breadsticks

Calories: 55, Net Carbs: 2.8 g, Fat: 19 g, Protein: 13 g

What you need:

1 1/2 cups of sunflower seeds

2 TSPs of pulverized psyllium husk

1/3 cup of cream cheese

2 cups of grated mozzarella cheese

1 large egg

1/2 TSP of sea salt

1 TSP of fresh rosemary

Steps:

1. Preheat your oven to the temperature of 400°F. Cover a cookie sheet using baking paper or utilize a non-stick baking mat.
2. Using the food processor on high, pound the sunflower seeds till it becomes ground into flour.
3. In the big bowl, you need to stir the psyllium husk, sunflower seed flour, and chopped rosemary & mix together. Set to the side.
4. Use a double boiler on high or medium heat in order to let the cream cheese and mozzarella cheese melt together.
5. Combine all the stirred ingredients together and incorporate completely.
6. Spoon out heaping TSPs of the dough and roll by hand into

small sticks. Put it into a prepared baking sheet. Slice horizontal lines into them with the spatula or back of a knife.
7. Heat for 12 minutes in the stove and sprinkle with rosemary and sea salt.

Tricks and Tips:

- These Rosemary sea salt breadsticks will store nicely in a sealed container for 5 days. They will soften slightly over that period of time.
- This recipe is ideal for the person who is allergic to nuts as it uses sunflower seeds ground into flour. This will also work as a substitute for any almond or coconut flour in these recipes.

Zucchini Breadsticks

Total Prep & Cooking Time: 40 minutes

Makes: 30 Breadsticks

Calories: 55, Net Carbs: 2.8 g, Protein: 12 g, Fat: 14 g

What you need:

1 cup of mozzarella cheese

1 large of shredded zucchini

Salt & pepper, to taste

1/2 cup cheddar cheese—shredded

1 T. of almond flour

1 T. of oregano

Chopped coriander

2 large eggs

Steps:

1. Set your oven to a temperature of 350°F. You have to cover the baking sheet using "parchment paper", or you can simply use a silicone-based baking mat.
2. Put almond flour & eggs in a big bowl & combine them well. Then add the mozzarella cheese, salt, pepper, and oregano and mix together well.
3. Cut the ends of the zucchini off and discard along with the seeds. Using long strokes, shred the zucchini using the standup grater's large holes.
4. Put the shredded zucchini on a tea towel and twist to make sure the excess juice is removed.
5. Fold in the shredded zucchini to the batter & thoroughly stir it

till incorporated fully.
6. Pour the dough into the lined baking sheet and ensure it is spread across as uniformly as possible.
7. Put the breadsticks in the stove for 20 minutes and dust the breadsticks with cheddar cheese and coriander.
8. Put the breadsticks on broil for 5 additional minutes until the cheese is melted.
9. Set them aside for 3 minutes and slice with a sharp knife or pizza cutter.
10. Serve warm and enjoy!

Tricks and Tips:

- It is especially important to ensure the zucchini has as much moisture removed as possible. If there is still water present in the zucchini when it is added to the batter, the breadsticks will result in being too soggy affecting them holding together properly.
- Do not fret if you did not get it right the first time. Simply turn the temperature of the oven up to 375°F and keep an eye on the dish. Pull the baking sheet out of the oven when they have the golden crispy tops. Then proceed to let them cool for 3 minutes before cutting them into breadsticks.

Index for the Recipes

Chapter 4: Muffin Recipes

Blueberry Muffins
Chocolate Chip Muffins
Cinnamon Sugar Muffins
Double Chocolate Muffins
Egg Muffins
French Toast Muffins
Pumpkin Cream Cheese Muffins
Raspberry Lemonade Muffins

Chapter 5: Cookie Recipes

Chocolate Sea Salt Cookies
Coconut Cookies
Florentine Cookies
Nutty Cookies
Nutty Chocolate Chip Cookies
Oatmeal Cookies
Oreo Cookies
Vanilla Crescent

Chapter 6: Bun and Bagel Recipes

Bun Recipes:
Dinner Rolls
Hawaiian Sweet Rolls
Mini Buns
Sesame Buns

Bagel Recipes:
Blueberry Cheesecake Bagels
Cheese Bagels
Jalapeno Bagels
Pizza Bagel Bites

Chapter 7: Bread Loaf Recipes

Blueberry Bread
Cauliflower Bread
Cheese and Bacon Bread
Hearty Seeded Bread
Pumpkin Bread
Quick Low-Carb Bread
Savory Bread

Chapter 8: Pizza Crust and Breadstick Recipes

Pizza Crust Recipes:
Coconut Flour Pizza Crust
Fathead Pizza Crust
Zero Carb Pizza Crust

Breadstick Recipes:
Cauliflower Breadsticks
Cheese Breadsticks
Garlic Breadsticks
Italian Breadsticks
Rosemary Sea Salt Breadsticks
Zucchini Breadsticks

CPSIA information can be obtained
at www.ICGtesting.com
Printed in the USA
BVHW061511181121
621928BV00002B/33